PLANTAR FASCIITIS HAS THE WRONG NAME

FitOldDog's Whole-Body Approach To Curing Your Nociceptive Foot Pain

DR. KEVIN T. MORGAN, BVSC, PHD, DIPACVP

It ain't what you don't know that gets you into trouble. It's what you know for sure that just ain't so.
– Mark Twain

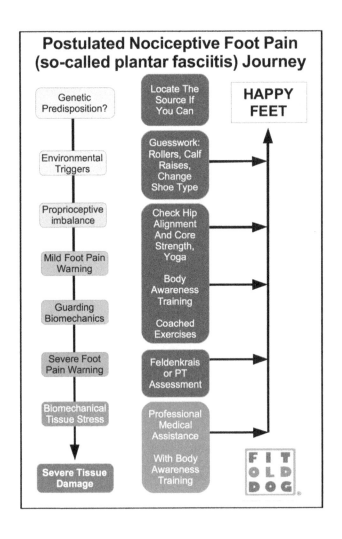

DEDICATION

This book was inspired by, and is dedicated to, the memory of Drs. Ignaz Semmelweis and John Snow, who provided light in the darkness of arrogance and ignorance, respectively.

PROLOGUE

One Case Solved

It took eight years of research for Tom to work out what is going on with acute morning (runner's) heel pain aka plantar fasciitis.

It's not confined to runners, by the way. This kind of heel pain is associated with pregnancy, being overweight, overtraining, poor posture, inadequately supportive shoes, and many other factors. But they all appear to be secondary to a primary cause.

Tom's online research, using patient surveys, demonstrated that almost all advertised treatments either (a) heal the heel pain, (b) have no effect, or (c) even make it worse. This includes the ministrations of podiatrists and doctors.

Tom's research, as presented in this book, was designed to track down the root cause of *so-called plantar fasciitis*.

THIS LED TO A RAPID CURE FOR ELISE

Elise is a runner who lives in Tom's neighborhood. She is in her late twenties, and boy, can she run! She heard from a friend, of Tom's interest in plantar fasciitis, and asked for his advice. Elise explained, *The plantar fasciitis heel pain in my right foot has been ruining my runs for* months. *The pain is worse when I run downhill, rather than uphill. Orthotics also made it worse.*

Tom instructed Elise to do as follows:

"It's important to cure this, before you do real damage to your feet or elsewhere in your legs and hips. The trick is to change the way you move. There are many ways to do this, such as changing shoe type, modifying your stride as you run, or studying body movement.

When the pain occurs, stop and stretch your hamstrings. Carry out a regular program of rolling your calves. Focus your stretching routine on your hips and hamstrings. Combine this with gentle strength training, including single-leg calf raises as they condition your legs, hips, and core. Do everything on both sides of your body."

Tom reminded Elise that stretching is a conversation you have with your body, not something you *do* to your body.

One week later, Elise told Tom that she had managed to run 16 miles, pain free. She was delighted, in her subdued, unassuming way.

Elise said, *I noticed a huge improvement when I rolled and stretched both my hips and hamstrings. I also used a Lacrosse ball to stretch deep muscles in my hips. I incorporated lunges before and after running, to stretch quads and hip flexors. The pain resolved after a week with your stretching and strengthening program. For the first time, I noticed that I had more tightness in my right hip muscles, including the pyriformis, than on the left side.*

Elise's report provided Tom with both encouragement and a mine of information. She is still enjoying long-distance running, pain free. Tom recently saw her steaming up a local hill, and wished he could run that well.

Tom doesn't have great resources, but he loves these little successes. They keep his investigations going.

Does this mean what worked for Elise will work for you?

Not necessarily, but if you understand the underlying mechanisms of your heel pain, you will be on the right track. Tom's been working to unravel this mystery for years. Here's his story, which is the source of the treatment strategy recommended in chapter ten.

FOREWORD

Pain is an action signal, not a damage meter.
– Todd Hargrove, *Guide to Better Movement* (2014)

Tom, a veterinarian, became a late-life triathlete, suffered excruciating pain, and made a surprising discovery about the common foot condition doctors call *plantar fasciitis*. Due to unexpected circumstances, he became obsessed with solving the cause of this heel pain. Tom is not only a veterinarian, he is also a widely published research pathologist.

Pathology is the study of the nature of disease.

Tom suffered his first bout of severe heel pain when he was in his sixties.

Damn, that hurt, he thought. *Like a knife stabbed in my heel the minute my foot touches the floor in the morning. Ruined my runs, too!*

A doctor (and Google) told Tom he had *plantar fasciitis*.

The doctor prescribed a pain killer, and told him to return if it didn't abate. She also told Tom that he might need an injection of cortisone into his heel. Tom didn't take the pain killers or return. Instead, he did what any research pathologist would do: He investigated theories about the underlying cause and recommended treatments.

Tom tried "the night splint." This costly device locks on your lower leg in a way that pulls on your calf muscles. This assumes that the heel pain is due to tight calves. Didn't do any good for Tom's heel pain, or his sleep for that matter. Then he tried rolling the sole of his foot on a frozen water bottle. He tested over-the-counter shoe inserts. Then did odd movements, recommended on a YouTube video. Then he consulted a chiropractor, followed by expensive orthotics prescribed by a podiatrist. The morning heel pain persisted.

Finally, his eldest son, Nick, said, "Dad, why don't you try rollers, they're great. You probably have tight calves."

Tom undertook a course of calf-rolling. He added single-leg calf raises to his routine, to strengthen his calves, as *"Underneath tightness, lies weakness."* The morning (and running) heel pain went away within a few weeks.

So Tom wrote a blog post, describing what had happened.

A few months later, Nick, said, "Dad, you should see this email I received the other day, from my friend Ryan, in Dallas."

It went like this:

Hey Dude, after 4 months of enduring the pain of plantar fasciitis and following all the wrong instructions from friends (rest, nighttime boot, ice, etc), I came across some old guy's blog post and it's been nothing short of amazing. Within a few days, I saw results and was walking my dog again without fear and I'm up to 4 mile run now. I just need to get in shape for that marathon. By the way, that old guy turned out to be your dad. Cheers, Ryan

This led to the publication of an e-book, *FitOldDog's Plantar Fasciitis Treatment*, written in collaboration with Tom's remarkable body-movement teacher, Rebecca Amis Lawson. They thought they'd solved the mystery of so-called *plantar fasciitis*.

TOM HAD A LOT MORE TO LEARN

As a pathologist, Tom was left with a niggling doubt: *Why call it plantar fasciitis, when the pain was all around my heel, and not confined to the plantar fascia? And why are so many different treatments advertised on Google? And why is there no consensus on the underlying cause? This would make a great research project for a graduate student or post-doc.*

Tom had retired from science. He no longer had a lab, staff or a budget. He still wondered whether he might tackle the problem.

CHAPTER ONE: QUESTIONING THE OBVIOUS

If a medical professional says you have *plantar fasciitis*, you have a puzzle to solve. No one, not even your doctor, can be sure of the best solution. So, beware!

The tools you will need:

- Your powers of observation.
- Your ability to question the obvious.
- Your willingness to experiment, using the strategic approach provided in this book (see chapter ten, if you can't wait).

The best tool in your toolbox is your mind. An open mind. Before you move on, here's a little test of your tools, to get you thinking like a scientist when it comes to your heel pain.

Two-hundred and thirty seven people, who claimed to have *plantar fasciitis,* responded to one of Tom's online research surveys. The most frequently reported treatment was changing shoe type. This gave the following result:

Heel Pain Response to Changing Shoe Type (% of respondants)	
Improved	49.48
No Change	39.18
Worse	7.22
Not Tested	4.12

What does this mean to you?

What questions does it raise in your mind?

Furthermore, here are the types of shoes people claimed had helped their symptoms, from 161 survey respondents. What does this mean?

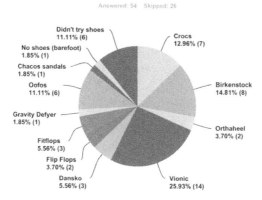

There are clues in these data. That is what science is about. Finding, questioning, interpreting and testing clues. Here's a short story Tom used to tell his students, as they learned to interpret their research results.

THE FLEA

A boy was walking along the street with his friend. Suddenly, his friend put his hand in his pocket, and said, "Do you want to see the flea I trained to jump on command?"

"Sure" said the boy. Of course he did. This was interesting.

His friend places a little black flea in the palm of his left hand and it just sits there.

Then he says, "Jump!" And the flea jumps clear across to land in his friend's right hand. The boy is amazed. But his friend says, "You haven't seen anything, yet." He reaches across and pulls one leg off of the flea. Then he repeats, "Jump." And again, on command, the flea jumps back to his left hand. The boy is really impressed, but his friend says, "You haven't seen anything yet." He repeats the jumping process until the flea has only one leg. Jump! And bravely the abused flea leaps the gap to the other hand.

Finally, the boys friend removes the last leg from the flea, and issues his command. Jump! JUMP! JUMP!

The flea refuses to obey.

What does this prove?

It's obvious.

When you remove all the legs from a flea, it goes deaf.

This is a silly joke, but it's a salutary tale, when it comes to the challenge of data interpretation.

Pain in your heel? Must be a problem in your heel. Probably inflamed. An injection of anti-inflammatory cortisone into your heel should fix it!

CHAPTER TWO: THE NATURE OF SCIENCE

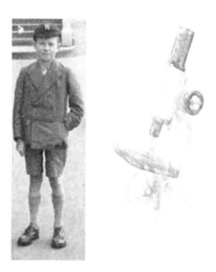

Tom aged twelve, and his beloved microscope.

NOT ALL READERS ARE SCIENTISTS

If you are a scientist just skip this chapter, if you wish. Then again, not all scientists think alike, and you might not like Tom's approach. If so, read on! The purpose of this chapter is to provide a glimpse into the mind of Tom, a scientist who loves science. Tom enjoyed studying biology ever since he was a kid.

THE SCIENTIFIC METHOD: *Principles and procedures for the systematic pursuit of knowledge involving the recognition and formulation of a problem, the collection of data through observation and experiment, and the formulation and testing of hypotheses.*

– Merriam-Webster Online Dictionary

To Tom the problem was clear, "What is the underlying cause of the condition doctors call plantar fasciitis, and how is it best treated?" Tom was quite familiar with collecting data, and he went about it in a number of ways, as you will see.

However, there is more to science than the linear logical strategy defined above. Science is full of surprises, guesswork, intuitions, hunches, epiphanies and persistence in the face of resistance. The real challenge is to question the obvious. This is difficult, as the obvious is hard to spot. Our brains ignore it as just the way things are!

QUESTIONING THE OBVIOUS

It's obvious that doctors know what they're doing. Right? They are highly trained in the treatment of pain. As Tom cogitated, he remembered the doctor saying he might need a heel injection. *A what? What was she thinking?* This raised Tom's suspicions concerning whether this doctor really understands the structure and function of the heel. As a medical professional, the thought of a heel injection horrified Tom. His thoughts went like this:

The connective tissue of the heel isn't a random blob of collagen and elastin. It's a complex living structure that responds to load. Interactions with the ground, as we move, subject it to shear and compression forces. This creates patterns of strain throughout the collagen/elastin network, thus sculpting the structure of the molecular cross-links and alignments within this critical support system. Jabbing needles in there is like chucking paint on a work of art, or jamming a spanner (monkey wrench) in the works. Plus there's the risk of infection.

Tom was suspicious, the first step in the scientific method. Clearly, more thought was needed.

Epiphany

An intuitive grasp of reality through something (such as an event) usually simple and striking.

– Merriam-Webster Online Dictionary

In science, flashes of insight are critical opportunities. Such epiphanies are generally the result of years of cogitation and experimentation. Here's a story demonstrating how scientific epiphany works.

Sunday, 8:30 a.m., 1995

The phone rings. *Tom, it's Jim. I have the answer.*

Jim is a research chemical engineer. He'd been a visiting scientist in Tom's fluid mechanics lab for about six months. For the past 12 years, Tom had struggled to solve a problem. *Why were lesions in the noses of rats, induced by inhaled formaldehyde, so precisely cut? With such sharp margins. Normal cells directly adjacent to completely destroyed tissue. You'd expect a fuzzy margin of less affected tissue! How could this be?* Many scientists, from biochemists to mathematicians, had worked with Tom on this question, which involved toxicology, biochemistry, physical chemistry, and fluid dynamics.

Tom's question intrigued Jim. Tom and Jim tried one thing after another, some weird, some more pedestrian. All led to blind alleys.

Then the phone call.

Jim (Excited): Fill the flow tank with dilute developer. Place exposed X-ray film on the floor, and …

Tom (Now wide awake): Got it. Tom hung up and rushed to his lab.

This trip led to the most remarkable image Tom had ever seen in his flow tank. The tank's design was based on one created by Dr. Steven Vogel at Duke University to study the swimming mechanics of squid.

The image appeared slowly, over about ten minutes. The flow tank motor hummed in the background, as dilute hydroquinone solution flowed through the tank and over the black x-ray film. This flow created a steady, but complex flow field over the surface of the film. The rate of development of the depended on the rate at which developer reached the film. This rate is influenced by the way the flowing fluid interacts with the floor of the tank.

Think of a stream, cutting away the bank here, doing nothing there. In the case of the flow tank, there were two things influence exposure of the film to the developer. Flow patterns (convection) and rate of diffusion of hydroquinone towards the film. It was like watching a photo develop, downstream of the microtome chuck that Tom had used to hold the x-ray film in place. But there was no photo, as all of the film was exposed.

Jim's insightful experiment revealed the pattern of the rate of exposure of the x-ray film to the developer chemicals. It was just like exposure of the nose to formaldehyde in air, which also involves both convection and diffusion.

The odd piece of metal set up a complex flow field in the developer, above the film. This flow field, of vortices, streamlines, and eddies, was painting the picture as silver grains were removed from the film film. Fine details emerged, including sharp cuts, just like those in the nose of a rat that Tom had seen under a microscope in 1981!

This fluid flow 'photo' was consistent with the hypothesis that the distribution of formaldehyde-induced lesions in the nose of the rat (and surely humans, too), is due to boundary layer structure in the air phase, where complex airflow fields are present adjacent to the lining of the nose, during inspiration.

Sound boring? Well, scientists get really excited about such things!

One blind alley after another had been tested and abandoned. Tom's formaldehyde research journey cost millions of dollars, spawned many publications, even a movie, and opened career paths for several young scientists. The information-packed image in his flow tank that day was the result of work that spanned many years, and involved multiple scientific disciplines. Overall, it was solved that day, by Jim's remarkable but simple experiment.

Back to pain

That's how science works, and that's how Tom's worked for the last eight years to solve the mystery of so-called plantar fasciitis. First, Tom needed to study the nature of pain. Apparently, veterinarians receive more pain education than do doctors, and Tom has learned a lot about this mysterious beast.

CHAPTER THREE: PAIN PUZZLES

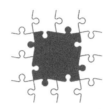

Puzzle

transitive verb

To offer or represent to (someone) a problem difficult to solve or a situation difficult to resolve : challenge mentally; also : to exert (oneself, one's mind, etc.) over such a problem or situation they puzzled their wits to find a solution.

– Merriam-Webster Online Dictionary

It's the summer of 2001, and Tom, in his late 50s, is watching the Lake Placid Ironman race. Lake Placid is a quiet little town in up-state New York, not far from the Canadian border. Well, it's quiet unless the Ironman race is on, which happens every July. A full Ironman race includes a 2.4-mile swim, 112-mile bike ride, and a 26.2-mile marathon, all in one day. Are these people crazy?

Three thousand athletes of all ages have stationed themselves in the beautiful, crystal clear water of Mirror Lake. The water reflects a cloudless blue sky and the breathtaking Adirondack mountains. It's a perfect backdrop to a perfect day. Cool, a light breeze, low humidity. What could be better?

The crazy people in the lake are awaiting the starter's gun. It goes off at 7:00 am, on the dot. Sitting in a cold lake is not Tom's idea of fun. The thought makes him shiver. Tom looks down on the water from a grassy bank. One of the white, pink and blue swim caps is on the head of his youngest son, Nigel, a good-looking, tall, muscular young man. A remarkable athlete.

Tom is a proud father and spectator. The energy of the competitors and the excitement of the crowd sucks him in, as he watches the swim start. Three thousand bobbing heads turn into a churning mass of arms and legs. Each swimmer must force his or her way through the maelstrom. To Tom, a swimmer and water-polo player in his youth, this looks pretty dicey for the weaker swimmers, at least.

At the swim-finish-to-bike-transition, Tom watches Nigel head out on his triathlon bike, giving his dad a friendly wave as he goes by. Nigel looks completely relaxed, unfazed by the 2.4-mile swim, which he completed in less than an hour. He'd told his dad that the swim was the easy part. By the early afternoon, Tom is stationed in an ideal spot to watch Nigel return on his bike from the Adirondacks, and to start the run.

The last leg of an Ironman is a grueling marathon. In less than 10 hours from the swim start, Nigel makes the final turn to the finish line, at the high school stadium. Tom leans on a retaining fence, a hundred yards from the finish. It's a noisy, energetic place, full of family and friends, everyone jockeying for a better view as the athletes enter the stadium to deafening applause.

Then, from the loudspeakers comes the announcement: *"NIGEL MORGAN, YOU ARE AN IRONMAN."*

I'd like to do that, Tom thinks. And he does. Takes him ten years.

On that July day, in 2001, leaning over that fence, little did Tom know what he was letting himself in for. If there were any weak links in Tom's physical or mental chains, the Ironman would reveal them. He was pretty fit for an older guy, but he was no Ironman: five foot six, built more like a wrestler than a cyclist or runner, with skinny legs and a big head. A nerd, not an athlete.

Tom's decision, made in the heat of the moment, was to take him on a painful journey. He was about to learn a great deal about physical pain, including heel pain.

Swimming

As an enthusiastic water polo player, in his youth, Tom knew how to sprint in the pool. But long-haul, open-water swimming? Not so much. Then he discovered the Total Immersion Swimming Technique, created by real long-distance swimmers, who swim tens of miles in the open ocean. It's about balance and endurance, not speed, as is the Ironman, when you undertake it in your sixties, seventies and beyond.

The effect of Total Immersion on Tom's swimming efficiency was remarkable. It also led to him to understand the critical role of balance in body movement, whether swimming, biking or running. After he'd conditioned his body in the pool, Tom's long-distance swims were up to snuff. This lesson would prove important to his later studies of "plantar fasciitis," which Tom would come to call nociceptive foot pain (NFP). But that's getting ahead of the story.

Poor balance, in the water or on dry land, leads to constant, generally imperceptible corrections.

OK! First part worked out. Only took a year or so.

Cycling

Tom cycled a lot as a youngster. One hundred and twelve miles through the Adirondack Mountains would be tough, but doable. For the next few years, Tom biked thousands of miles, with a cycling partner, Rory, an experienced cyclist. It took several years for Rory to knock Tom's cycling into any kind of shape.

Tom's success on the bike was revealed by a comment from Rory, about sixty miles into a long ride. "Say, Tom, let's do this extra twenty-mile loop. It's one I like, and it'll bring our distance up to about a hundred miles for the day. What do you think?"

Tom agreed, and Rory pulled away. All Tom could do was hang close to Rory's rear wheel. The twenty miles were a grueling battle to not be dropped, as cyclists say. As Rory and Tom reached the end of the extra loop, Rory spit out, "You fu**er!" Rory then admitted he'd been trying to drop Tom the whole time. Tom felt both dog-tired and triumphant on the ride home.

Competitive cycling is very much about mastering pain. You soon learn the difference between good and bad pain. Good pain leads to conditioning and better performance. Bad pain indicates risk of injury. It takes a while, and a few injuries, to recognize the difference. Furthermore, balance is critical for safe bike handling and performance. For cyclists, rule number one, *keep the rubber side down!*

Running

Tom was starting to develop a level of Ironman fitness and skill. This was becoming a way of life. Now to add the running piece. *Shouldn't be too bad*, Tom told himself. Little did he know!

Tom hadn't enjoyed running in his youth. His legs lacked the stamina for it. Mild rickets as a toddler, due to poor nutrition, led to weak bones and joints, one of the effects of World War II. Tom was born in England in 1943, eighteen months before the end of the war. Even though his Mum did a great job, food, especially good food, was scarce for the first ten years of his life. War is hard on kids.

War and rickets aside, you can't complete an Ironman without learning how to run a marathon on tired legs. He took lessons from his triathlete son. "You run like a loaf of bread," Nigel said, without explanation. It meant that Tom had no idea how to engage his whole body, while running. So he hired a coach and took running lessons, gradually increasing the distance.

Then trouble started. Every time he made it to five miles, his right knee expressed extreme distress. Pain! The deep, throbbing, "you-have-to-stop-running" kind. His coach recommended the gold standard of rest, ice and stretching, plus pain relief gel and a heating pad. Nothing helped.

Tom knew he had to fix this knee pain if he ever hoped to complete the 26.2-mile run segment of his Ironman dream. Over the next year, he tried everything he could think of to pass the five-mile running barrier. Finally, unable to solve the knee pain on his own, he sought professional medical help. As he had a well-paid job and health insurance, money wasn't a major issue. But where to seek advice?

His coach suggested a sports physician. Nigel recommended his friend Dave, a talented triathlete and sports physician, with considerable experience of running problems. Dave applied ultrasound to Tom's knee. This he combined with running analysis videos and X-rays. They worked on relaxing Tom's leg muscles, along with strength training. But after weeks of work still no improvement!

In despair, Tom moved on. Several fellow athletes suggested a chiropractor, so he gave it a go. Two well-known chiropractors later, Tom still could not pass the five-mile run barrier. Knee pain stopped him around five miles, every time.

"How about a sports massage therapist," one friend suggested. He went to a masseuse, Carolyn, who works with the UNC-Chapel Hill track team. In the process, Tom learned a great deal about tight muscles. He also experienced how painful and effective sports massage can be. In spite of Carolyn's remarkable massage skills, nothing changed.

Was Tom's Ironman dream becoming an expensive nightmare?

To keep a long story short, there was no improvement. Not with Yoga, kinesiology, or acupuncture. Nor with several podiatrists and their expensive orthotics, and two physical therapists. Each of these experienced professionals scratched their heads, then presented their bills for payment.

A second sports medicine physician diagnosed an inflamed bursa in Tom's knee, and injected the anti-inflammatory drug cortisone into the bursa. It hurt a bunch, but made no difference in Tom's running.

A year gone by, over three thousand dollars spent, and nothing to show for it.

There was a bright side, however. Tom gained insights into the nature of a wide range of physical therapy disciplines. Later, he would benefit from this experience. But what about the Ironman?

Moshe to the rescue

One sunny day, Tom was wandering around his favorite coffee shop and health-food market, when he ran into Karen, an attractive and soft-spoken woman. "Hi, Tom, what's up?" *she said.* "Haven't seen you since I left science, several years ago."

Karen informed Tom that she'd abandoned molecular biology to teach the Feldenkrais Method, a method invented by Moshe Feldenkrais, after he suffered a serious knee injury while playing soccer. Moshe used his approach to return to his beloved soccer. "The Feldenkrais Method is now employed all over the world," Karen explained. "It's used to help people recover from injuries. Both athletes and musicians use Feldenkrais to improve their performance."

Tom said, "That's interesting. Do you think you can you fix my running-induced knee pain?" Tom told Karen about his litany of attempted cures, and she said that she would be happy to give it a go. The following week, Tom arrived at Karen's house, expecting another failure for his $70.

First, Karen asked him to walk around her home office, while she watched. Then she said, "Stand in front of me, relax, and sway from side to side."

Tom did as instructed.

Tom's understanding of the pains of body movement were about to change forever. Karen spoke these magic words:

"Tom, did you know that when you sway to the left your body remains straight? When you sway to the right, your shoulders rotate a little. Your right shoulder moves forward a few millimeters."

He looked down, and there it was! *But what did it mean*?

"Have you had any serious accidents in the past?"

"Well, I did have a motorcycle wreck about forty years ago, which broke my right ankle." He couldn't imagine what that would have to do with anything.

"I suspect that you're guarding, or locking, that damaged right ankle. This forces your body to turn around your hips, as you sway to the right. Do you have more trouble balancing on your right leg?"

The jig was up!

He'd been locking that right ankle ever since a motorbike wreck in his teens. Guarding, or psychosomatic tension, protects damaged tissues in the short-term. If it becomes a habit, however, guarding or locking can lead to problems. Tom had effectively immobilized that painful ankle to protect it after the motorcycle wreck. He was still doing it more than forty years later. This impaired the movement efficiency of his right leg. It also made it hard for him to balance on that leg.

Balancing on one leg requires constant fine adjustments of the ankle to stay upright. It would appear that balance is also critical for effective running. Karen concluded that this strain was causing the pain in his knee, after several miles of running.

It had no effect on Tom's walking or cycling, but running is less forgiving, as is balancing on one leg. His knee pain was due to an issue with his ankle, believe it or not! And Karen had diagnosed it by simply observing the way he moved! Critically, she hadn't assumed that pain in his knee was due to a primary problem in his knee.

Two millimeters rotation of his shoulders, less than the thickness of a couple of dimes. This tiny movement revealed the cause of Tom's running pain. It directed Tom to pay attention to his ankle, his accident history, and the study of body movement. It also raised Tom's awareness of the critical nature of balance when running.

Fixing his ankle stiffness fixed Tom's running-induced knee pain. The pain was an action signal, all right. The action needed wasn't in his knee, but in his ankle.

Pain as an Action Signal

If pain is an action signal, not a damage meter, what action did Tom need to take? It was simple! Tom had to stop locking that ankle, and return it to its normal flexibility. This involved breaking down scar tissue from the wreck, and improving joint mobility. Tom followed the advice of Bruce Buley, an excellent physical therapist.

The work involved using a hand towel wrapped around his foot, to twist it to the outside. This stretched his ankle away from the area of scarring and tightness on the inside. Tom's ankle had been caught between an incoming car and the metal kickstart lever of his heavy motorbike (OUCH!) all those years ago.

Bruce also gave Tom a copy of a remarkable book *Running With the Whole Body*, by Jack Heggie. It's based on the Feldenkrais Method. Along with *Chi Running*, by Danny Dreyer, this method created Tom's eventual low-impact running style. Otherwise, Tom would never have qualified for the Boston Marathon, at age 66, in 2008. All part of his Ironman training.

Within weeks of his meeting with Karen, Tom was running pain-free for ten miles or more. He went on to complete the Lake Placid Ironman five times, in his late sixties and early seventies. The fourth to last time Tom completed this race, it saved him from an early death, as it led to his detection of a massive abdominal aortic aneurysm, about to burst. But that's another story.

Fixing heel pain

Tom's knee pain story played a critical role in his understanding of the nature of pain. Tom had learned that the interpretation of pain is not always a simple matter. He suspected that it's always trying to tell us something, but the message can be hard to puzzle out.

CHAPTER FOUR: DATA COLLECTION BEGINS

Tom was in his favorite running store, trying on a pair of zero-rise, large-toe-box running shoes. He was also quizzing fellow athletes and staff about whether they'd suffered from *plantar fasciitis*.

JEFF'S STORY:

Jeff, who'd served Tom several times before, said, "I've been a runner all my life. I had plantar fasciitis once. It was a few years ago. Running's in my blood, I guess. I was having a great season, when I suddenly developed a horrible heel pain. It was worst on getting out of bed in the morning and when I ran. It really messed up my run. I'd end up hobbling within a few miles.

The sports doc said I had plantar fasciitis. I tried lots of treatments, but nothing worked.

I'd already signed up for a 100-mile run, and was pretty excited about it, but the foot pain was crippling me. I thought, to hell with it, I'll do the run anyway. So I did!

Yes! I was nervous.

I set off, and had a horrible time for the first 60 miles. My heel hurt but I pushed through it. Long-distance running involves plenty of pain, either way.

Then, surprise, surprise. Around mile 60, my heel pain vanished. I just noticed that it wasn't there anymore. That was several years ago, and I haven't had heel pain since!"

Based on this story, you might be tempted to run - or walk - through your own pain. Not so fast. Read on.

Anne's Story

It was the first day of a triathlon training camp, and about fifteen athletes, including Tom, were sitting in a circle. Dave, the head coach, said, "I'd like each of you to tell your most severe training injury story. Let's see what we can learn. *I learned that you should hang onto the bike when you're hit by an SUV!"*

Dave was in a wheelchair, recovering from a serious bike wreck - a constant hazard when training on the road. Anne, a tall blond, about 25, slim, very fit, and shy, was clearly an excellent athlete.

"I was training for an important race, when I developed a horrible heel pain in both feet." Anne said. "It was really bad in the morning, but it never went away all day. A sports doc said I had plantar fasciitis, and recommended that I stop running for a while. He said there was a risk of seriously injuring my plantar fascia.

But I continued my training anyway. You know how it is! I was doing a steady 10-mile out and back in our neighborhood, when both plantar fascias ripped in half. I collapsed in unimaginable pain, and my neighbor found me and carted me off to the hospital. The same sports doc came to see me, but he didn't say I told you so! He's a good doctor, and I trust him.

I ended up having surgery to repair my feet. With intense physical therapy, it took me over a year to walk normally, and another year to start running.

I'm finally back, but I'll never do that again."

Tom thought, *It can progress to involve the plantar fascia, but only in extreme cases.*

Then he wondered, *How did Jeff fix his heel pain by running, and Anne tore up her feet doing essentially the same thing? Running through the pain. This doesn't sound like inflammation.*

IT WAS TIME FOR TOM TO FIND MORE DATA.

First he went to Facebook. People love to talk about their problems on Facebook. Tom soon found several sites dedicated to plantar fasciitis. He read hundreds of stories about people's frustrations and successes with their heel pain. Tom asked people questions, to get a feel for the condition. He then created tables of data from comments on the effectiveness of different treatments.

PEOPLE WERE STARTING TO BUY TOM AND REBECCA'S EBOOK.

Some found the approach in the book helpful. The book was a good start, but Tom wanted to help more people by improving his Internet marketing skills. He asked his friend Walter, a businessman in England, for advice. "Create an attractive visual." Walter said. "Moving images, an interactive diagram, or even a marketing video."

Tom had no experience with such things, and no budget, apart from retirement savings. He looked for something he could afford, and soon came across an interactive mapping system. This allowed Tom to build a picture of the available plantar fasciitis causes and treatments, with interactive links. The viewer simply clicked on a link to be taken to the relevant information or advertisement.

Tom spent the next few months building his map, and in the process he learned a great deal about the plantar fasciitis treatment market place. Here's a picture of this map.

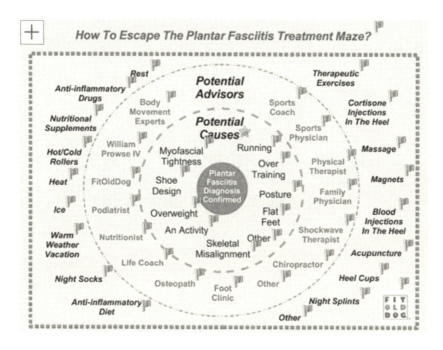

Go to limberfeet.com to see the interactive version on the Internet. Then "mouse over" the flags to see the embedded links. This is only a fraction of the information available.

On reviewing his work, Tom was reminded of Occam's Razor.

OCCAM'S RAZOR OR THE LAW OF PARSIMONY

Occam's Razor is a problem-solving principle attributed to William of Ockham (c. 1287–1347), an English Franciscan friar, scholastic philosopher and theologian. The principle can be summarized thus:

Among competing hypotheses, select the one that makes the fewest assumptions.

Tom wondered, *Can I find a common principle, amongst these treatments? If so, it should lead to an effective approach to curing this horrible heel pain that afflicts millions.*

CHAPTER FIVE: WEIRD DISEASE TREATMENTS
The black death, influenza and 'plantar fasciitis'

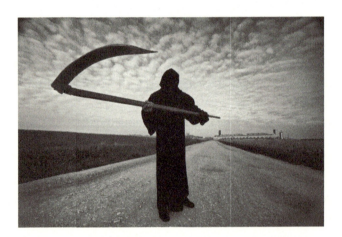

Therapeutics
A branch of medical science dealing with the application of remedies to diseases.

– Merriam-Webster Online Dictionary

While considering the weird array of plantar fasciitis treatments in his map, Tom's mind is carried back to his first year of veterinary school, in the 1960s. He remembered an interesting class on the history of medicine and therapeutics. Tom recalled treatments for the plague in medieval England.

476 TO 1492. THE BLACK DEATH KILLED MILLIONS

Plague, known as the black death, destroyed civilizations in medieval times. Entire towns were wiped out.

Imagine you were born in these times, and the plague arrived in town. You're scared to death, so you ask your priest, witch, or friend what to do. They might suggest you try one of the following:

- *Eat cooked onions.*
- *Eat some ten-year-old treacle.*
- *Swallow arsenic.*
- *Eat some crushed emeralds.*
- *Sit in the sewers.*
- *Stand between two big fires.*
- *Place herbs throughout your house, to keep the air clean.*
- *Bury your plague bodies in a holy well.*
- *Have a doctor drain the black bile from your blood.*
- *Pray for forgiveness. The black death is God's punishment for our sins.*

Of course, today we laugh at such suggestions. We know the plague is caused by bacteria (*Pasteurella pestis,* recently renamed *Yersinia pestis*). But that was ages ago. We're much wiser now.

PLAGUE TREATMENT TODAY:

<u>Cure</u>: We discovered the power of antibiotics to kill bacteria. This led to an easy treatment for the plague: Penicillin. Understanding the disease resulted in a reliable treatment.

<u>Prevention</u>: We now know that we contract this disease from rat fleas. This discovery led to prevention, through improved hygiene.

1918-1919. Influenza Killed Millions

Only 100 years ago, influenza killed tens of millions of people around the world. Here's a few treatments you might have been advised to try, at the time:

- *Wear a necklace of garlic (also keeps vampires away).*
- *Doctors recommend rectal injections of eucalyptus oil.*
- *Rub wormwood on your chest.*
- *Drink some pine tar.*
- *Put an onion in your room to absorb the flu, then throw the onion away.*
- *Smear steaming horse manure on your chest.*
- *Have some teeth pulled.*
- *Take strychnine.*

Flu Treatment Today:

Cure: The discovery that influenza is a viral infection led to the creation of antiviral drugs. Knowing the cause of the symptoms resulted in effective nursing strategies. Antibiotics prevent secondary infections. Decongestants offset airway blockage. Intravenous fluids prevent lethal dehydration and shock. *[handwritten: It's electrical!]*

Prevention: The flu virus comes to us via chickens and pigs. So animal health monitoring is in place. A vaccine is available. Furthermore, health protocols reduce spread of the virus from one person to another. These protocols include staying at home rather than going to work, not coughing around other people, wearing a face mask and washing your hands regularly.

2018. Plantar Fasciitis Afflicts Millions

You have horrible heel pain. Especially in the morning. Your doctor tells you it's *plantar fasciitis*. She suggests an injection of cortisone into your heel. You're not so sure about that, as you hate needles, and ask if you can think about it.

You Google *plantar fasciitis treatments*, and discover dozens of guaranteed cures.

- *Roll your foot on a frozen water bottle.*
- *Stretch your calves.*
- *Put magnets on your ankles.*
- *Take herbal supplements.*
- *Wear a special boot in bed, to stretch your calves.*
- *Get pregnant.*
- *Ask your doctor to give you an injection of platelet-rich plasma.*
- *Consider bare-foot running.*
- *Lose weight.*
- *Fix your collapsed arches.*
- *Try calf surgery for muscle/tendon lengthening (Strayer Technique) to reduce tension in the heel.*
- *Pray for it to go away.*

Sound familiar?

CHAPTER SIX: THE NAME OF A DISEASE CAN BE CRITICAL

It may determine the treatment

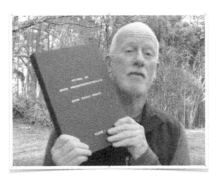

Tom published his doctoral thesis in 1975. The name he chose for the disease he studied turned out to be important.

Terminology: *The technical or special terms used in a business, art, science, or special subject.*

– Merriam-Webster Online Dictionary

The medical profession, under the auspices of the American Medical Association (AMA), controls the "official" naming of medical conditions, using:

- The name of the discoverer (e.g., Alzheimer's disease).
- The name of the first case diagnosed (e.g., Lou Gehrig's disease).
- Specific symptoms (e.g., sickle cell anemia).
- Assumptions about the nature of the disease (e.g., *"plantar fasciitis"*).

Once the name sticks, it's difficult to unstick it. It becomes fixed in textbooks, people's health records, statistical data tables, and people's minds. Not a trivial matter!

Tom Takes His PhD Examination

In 1975, Tom presented his doctoral research to the University of Edinburgh, Scotland, on *Ovine Polioencephalomalacia,* a disease of the nervous system of sheep. Tom's examining committee did not appreciate his using the term "polioencephalomalacia," as this was the name used in the United States. Post-war anti-American feeling was still running high in the British landscape.

Oversexed, overpaid and over here! was the sentiment in Great Britain at the time.

On examination day, Tom, in his late-twenties, all ginger hair and enthusiasm, arrived on time at the veterinary school. It's an intimidating building, which has now been converted into an art center and a very nice bar, decorated with veterinary paraphernalia.

Tom knocked on the door of the office assigned for his examination. On receiving no audible response, he entered a somber, wood lined, dimly lit room. Awaiting him were three inscrutable men. They wore serious expressions and the standard garb of veterinary research examiners: tweed jackets, conservative ties, and somewhat aggressive postures. They instructed Tom to take a seat. He wondered how this was going to go, given the mild hostility in the air.

Each member of his examining committee was well respected in his field: pathology, biochemistry, and bacteriology. Tom had employed these disciplines extensively in his doctoral research. Doctor of Philosophy (PhD) is a critical meal ticket in the world of research, and these three men held in their hands the power to grant or withhold that degree.

Tom's mother was tough; she had told him many times "You can fight city hall." Stand up to power, and you will earn their respect. Still, Tom was a little nervous.

On the front of Tom's two-volume thesis, in gold type, was the source of the tension. A copy lay in front of each examiner, with many paper markers inserted in each copy. At the time, the British name for the subject of Tom's thesis was *cerebro-cortical necrosis* (CCN). His defense opened with an immediate attack on his selection of the name *polioencephalomalacia,* a better name for this disease, in Tom's not-so-humble opinion.

Tom had opted for *polioencephalomalacia* because it was less misleading: the brain damage associated with this disease is not confined to the cerebral cortex. Tom's decision was based on logic, and on knowing more about the subject than anyone else in the room.

NOTE: When you sit for your PhD exam, you had better know much more about the subject of your thesis than your examination committee, or you'll be in trouble.

Tom did. Tom prevailed. On that day in 1975, he became Dr. Tom, BVSc, PhD!

This experience imbued him with a sense of the power of words and the importance of lexical semantics, especially when it comes to the names of diseases.

LEXICAL SEMANTICS: *The study of word meanings and word relations.*

When it comes to disease, words can determine the treatment, as it does in the case of so-called *plantar fasciitis.*

For example, the following was displayed on the Mayo Clinic website, as of this writing:

Plantar fasciitis (PLAN-tur fas-e-I-tis) is one of the most common causes of heel pain. It involves inflammation of a thick band of tissue that runs across the bottom of your foot and connects your heel bone to your toes (plantar fascia). Plantar fasciitis commonly causes stabbing pain that usually occurs with your first steps in the morning. As you get up and move more, the pain normally

decreases, but it might return after long periods of standing or after rising from sitting.
Plantar fasciitis is more common in runners. In addition, people who are overweight and those who wear shoes with inadequate support have an increased risk of plantar fasciitis.

This is the conventional wisdom of the day. Tom generally trusted the Mayo Clinic, and medical texts. Not this time, though. This misleading conventional wisdom on *plantar fasciitis* called to mind an experience Tom had as a young veterinarian.

1967, IN A SMALL VETERINARY PRACTICE IN BRISTOL, ENGLAND

As a young veterinarian, Tom was called out to a case of bovine uterine prolapse, his first time for this tricky problem in cows. Such prolapses involve the uterus falling out, inside out, after a calf is born. The uterus appears as a mass of wet, bright red, delicate tissue, covered in slime, hanging out of the rear end of a cow. It's often covered in dirt and straw. This mass of tissue is about one yard long and as much as a foot wide. It has to be returned to its normal place inside the cow. No easy task.

Tom remembered what he'd heard in class, and read in textbooks: *put it back (how?), stitch it in (into a straining and unhappy cow? You're joking!), and administer, oxytocin, to shrink the uterus back into place (fine).*

As Tom was leaving, John, one of the senior vets, asked, "Where are you off to, Tom?"

"A prolapse in a dairy cow."

"Is this your first case?"

Tom nodded To Tom's surprise, John told him to ignore the advice he'd received in vet school adding, "Those who can, do! Those who can't, teach. Follow me."

They went down a dark hallway to a cupboard, under some stairs. The older man scrabbled around in the cupboard and brought out a cardboard box. It contained a tea tray, a two-pound bag of sugar, a large bath towel, and a long, slender wine bottle.

"Here's what you do, Tom. Remember, if you break the uterus

while putting it back, the cow will probably die of peritonitis. Place the tray, covered with the spread-out towel, under the prolapse. This will require two helpers, if she's standing. And have a good person at her head, as she may try to turn and attack you, to protect her calf."

True. A couple of years later, a huge Friesian cow had nearly killed Tom. The farmer had been quick to distract the new mother, and just saved Tom from being gored.

"Pick off any straw, and rinse the prolapse with saline." John said. "Then, sprinkle on the sugar. This will suck a lot of fluid out of the swollen uterus, which will shrink by one third in about five minutes. Then, wrap it in the bath towel, and ease it back where it belongs. The towel will reduce the risk of you making a fatal hole with your fingers.

Once it's back in, push it as far as you can, as if you're straightening a sock that's inside out. If the uterus is too big for you to reach all the way, insert the wine bottle to increase your reach. This will allow you to return the uterus completely, so it won't slide right out again. Then give her the oxytocin, and that uterus will shrink down, to be firmly in place in minutes. And you're done."

It worked like a charm.

So much for conventional wisdom and textbook learning. There had been no mention of trays or wine bottles in Tom's veterinary training.

This experience later caused the much older Tom to be suspicious of the description of plantar fasciitis on the Mayo Clinic website.

IMPACT OF A NAME ON DISEASE TREATMENT

Tom considered the potential impact of the term *plantar fasciitis* on the minds of people attempting to treat the condition.

Plantar = the site of the connective tissue band that runs along the sole (plantar surface) of your foot. This part of the name draws one's attention towards the sole of foot, and away from possible causes elsewhere in the foot or more remotely in the body.

Remember Karen, the Feldenkrais instructor, and Tom's knee pain.

Fasciitis = inflammation of fascia (a dense connective tissue). Many people reach for anti-inflammatory drugs to treat *plantar fasciitis*.

However, Tom read one study (Lemont, Ammirati and Usen, 2003) that demonstrated there was no inflammation present in the plantar fascia in such cases. Tom's future studies were also consistent with the absence of inflammation in this condition. These authors stated that, "Serial corticosteroid injections into the plantar fascia should be reevaluated ... in light of their potential to induce plantar fascial rupture."

MATT'S STORY

Matt, a young photographer, was diagnosed with *plantar fasciitis* by his physician, who recommended a cortisone injection into his heel. It's possible to introduce infectious organisms whenever you penetrate the skin. That's exactly what happened to Matt. In fact, it was the worst possible infection, MRSA (*Methicillin Resistant Staphylococcus Aureus*). These bacteria are resistant to most antibiotics.

Matt ended up in the hospital because of an injection he never should have agreed to. He recovered, and is doing well, but he could have lost his foot. Matt's story contributed to Tom's frustration with misguided heel injections.

Why do medical professionals continue to administer these dangerous, and generally useless, injections? Tom wondered. *Don't they realize the nature of the delicate structures they're invading, willie-nilly?*

SUNDAY, JUNE 17TH, 2018, AT ABOUT 6:00 A.M.

While making his morning cup of tea, Tom had a flash of insight: An epiphany. *Those single-leg calf raises we put in FitOldDog's Plantar Fasciitis Treatment ebook years ago, were the first real clue. We just didn't know it. It's not about the effect of the exercise on the calf muscles, it's about how we move our bodies, especially in our hips. That's where to focus our attention: our hips. It could make sense of all those crazy treatments.*

Tom's a research scientist at heart. Things came together in his mind. As mentioned previously, flashes of insight are critical opportunities in science. Such epiphanies are generally the result of years of cogitation and experimentation. Suddenly it all made sense. A far cry from proof, but such insights can send people down the right path. This led to Tom's working hypothesis for the cause of the heel pain doctors call plantar fasciitis.

HYPOTHESIS

A supposition or proposed explanation made on the basis of limited evidence as a starting point for further investigation.

TOM'S WORKING HYPOTHESIS

So-called plantar fasciitis, acute morning heel pain or runner's heel pain, is a progressive condition. In its early stages, it is a nociceptive (pain-causing) response to body movement stresses. This pain is a warning of worse to come, including tissue damage, if you don't change the way you move! Hence, this foot pain is nociceptive in nature. Thus, Tom recommends the name, nociceptive foot pain (NFP).

NOCICEPTION

Sensory signaling indicating danger to the tissues of the body. It is one of the most important inputs contributing to pain.

– Todd Hargrove, Guide to Better Movement

RECOMMENDED NAME FOR SO-CALLED PLANTAR FASCIITIS:

Nociceptive Foot Pain (NFP).
Embrace this name and you will see no reason for dangerous heel injections or irreversible calf surgery. You will see no point in frozen water bottles, magnets or foot massage. However, you might think about how you move, develop more body-awareness, and focus on your hips as a possible source.

IT'S NOT EASY TO CHANGE PEOPLE'S MINDS

A respected biologist referred to Tom's research on *NFP (*'*plantar fasciitis*'*)* as *Junk science*. A podiatrist publicly stated that his work is *"Based on BS."* When Tom posted his nociceptive hypothesis on an open plantar fasciitis forum, the site managers banned him from the site within two hours with no explanation. The site was run by people who use calf surgery - the Strayer technique - to treat *NFP (*'*plantar fasciitis!*'*)*

Then Tom published a blogpost indicating that heel injections should be banned (see AthleteWithStent.Com). He gave five reasons, based on logic and observation. Almost immediately on a Facebook plantar fasciitis page, another podiatrist described Tom's work as *"The worst form of garbage."* Tom was then banned from that site, even though he remained polite and friendly. Such responses convinced Tom that he was onto something important.

Or why the vitriol?

The discipline of pathology is dedicated to unearthing the mechanisms of disease. Tom had been a research pathologist most of his professional life. Nothing is more fun to a pathologist than challenging ingrained and incorrect assumptions about the nature of a disease process.

In such debates it is critical to challenge the ideas with logic and data, and never to attack the person.

A SALUTARY TALE OF A POWERFUL OBSERVATION, IGNORED

Extracted from an article by <u>Rebecca Davis of North Carolina Public Radio</u>, January 12th, 2015.

The year 1846.
Our hero is Ignaz Semmelweis, a Hungarian doctor. He wondered why so many women in maternity wards were dying from puerperal fever, also known as childbed fever. He studied two maternity wards in the hospital. One staffed by male doctors and medical students and the other by female midwives. He counted the number of deaths on each ward.
He noticed that more women were dying in the doctors' clinic than in the

midwives' clinic. He tested things that may have been responsible. Whether the women delivered on their back or their side. Whether a priest passed through the ward, ringing a bell. Finally, Semmelweis hypothesized that there were cadaverous particles. Little pieces of corpse. That doctors and students were getting on their hands from the bodies they dissected. During delivery, these particles would get inside the women. Causing the women to develop the disease and die.

If Semmelweis' idea was correct, getting rid of those particles should cut down on the death rate.

He ordered medical staff to start cleaning their hands and instruments. With a chlorine solution. Chlorine, as we know today, is about the best disinfectant there is. He chose chlorine because he thought it would be the best way to get rid of any smell.

The rate of childbed fever fell dramatically.

You'd think everyone would be thrilled. Semmelweis had solved the problem! But they weren't thrilled. Did he think the doctors were responsible for transmitting childbed fever to their patients? And Semmelweis wasn't tactful. He berated people who disagreed with him and made some influential enemies. The doctors gave up the chlorine hand-washing, and Semmelweis lost his job.

Ignaz challenged the medical establishment to correct its thinking on the nature of a disease process. He paid the price. Maybe he could have been more tactful. But does tact really work against entrenched ideas and massive marketing budgets?

CHAPTER SEVEN: CHOLERA, PLANE CRASHES, AND BALANCE

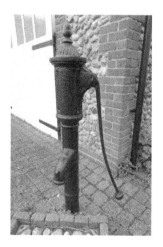

An old English water pump, much like that used by Dr. John Snow to discover the cause of cholera.

A single observation can lead to the discovery of the underlying cause of a disease. Here's Tom's favorite example, extracted from, *John Snow and the Broad Street Pump, On The Trail of an Epidemic*, by Kathleen Tuthill (UCLA, 2003).

Between 1831 and 1854, tens of thousands of people in England died of cholera. Doctor John Snow couldn't convince people that this disease spread in drinking water. He published an article in 1849 outlining his theory. But other doctors and scientists believed a 'miasma' in the atmosphere caused cholera.

Dr. Snow thought sewage near town wells was contaminating the water supply. In August of 1854, there was a terrible outbreak in Soho, a suburb of London. Dr. Snow, who lived near Soho, went to work to prove his theory that contaminated water was the source of cholera.

On September 7, 1854, Snow took his research to Soho's town officials. He convinced them to take the handle off the pump, making it impossible for the towns people to draw water. They were reluctant to do it, but they took the handle off as a trial, and the cholera outbreak stopped almost immediately.

In 1883, a German physician, Robert Koch, took the search for the cause of cholera a step further. He isolated the bacterium *Vibrio cholerae*, the "poison" Dr. Snow contended caused cholera. A simple test, removing the pump handle, had revealed the source of the disease. This single observation led to appropriate research. Knowing the cause resulted in ways to both prevent, and later to cure cholera, eventually saving the lives of millions.

A Heel Pain Epiphany

Back to 2014, and Tom, who was thinking about causes *versus* triggers. Tom had a second attack of NFP about a year after he dislocated (sub-luxated) his pelvis. This happened during a triathlon, as the result of a bike wreck. About ten months later, an osteopathic doctor put his pelvis back where it belonged. This chronic hip displacement had led to a pelvic soft tissue imbalance. Tom's hip muscles got tight on the left side, and stretched on the right. Such misalignments are trouble waiting to happen.

Then Tom developed a tightness in his right calf, on the opposite side to his tight hip. He was still training for Ironman, but was having trouble running, due to his tight right calf. In an attempt to rest that calf, he put arch supports in his running shoes. Then he ran two miles. Tom knew better, but he wanted to run. No fool like an old fool! But it felt so good!

The next morning, Tom suffered his worst case of heel pain yet. He had to crawl along the floor to get to the bathroom. The pain eased off during the day, to return in spades the next morning. Running also made it worse.

Tom wrote in his diary: "bike wreck -> subluxated pelvis -> tight left hip muscles -> tight right calf muscles -> arch supports plus run -> intense heel pain next morning."

This sequence of events reminded Tom of a story he'd read.

Plane Crashes

Tom recalled the following sentence, from Malcolm Gladwell's book, *Outliers, The Story of Success*:

"Plane crashes are much more likely to be the result of an accumulation of minor difficulties and seemingly trivial malfunctions." (page 183).

For instance, the pilot is overtired, the weather is bad, the plane's behind schedule, she/he has a new co-pilot and they are not comfortable with each other, then the co-pilot makes a trivial error of calculation, normally of no significance, but does not communicate the error to the pilot, the plane misses the runway, and crashes violently.

Aha! What if NFP results from a series of minor causes, the last one being the trigger or last straw? Tom thought, *Well, after a plane crash, they take the event apart to find out why. That's what we need to do with each new case of NFP.*

This might lead to an explanation for the data in the graph below, which shows that almost all the treatments examined, either (a) made things better, (b) had no effect, or (c) made things worse. Each case of heel pain, like each plane crash, is clearly unique to some degree.

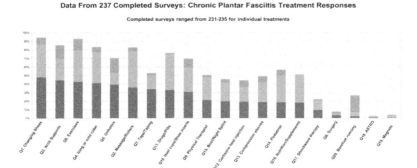

Data From 237 Completed Surveys: Chronic Plantar Faciitis Treatment Responses

Completed surveys ranged from 231-235 for individual treatments

■ Improved Symptoms   ■ No change   ■ Made it worse   ■ Not tested

These observations are not inconsistent with Tom's body movement hypothesis.

This time, Tom's heel pain was triggered by shoe inserts, and it hurt like crap. This one went on for about a year. Some expert (*physician heal thyself!*). Calf rolling and single-leg calf raises didn't do the trick. The pain lingered. Getting out of bed and running were miserable.

Instead of despairing, Tom saw his pain as an opportunity to do some first-hand research. So he watched the pain, to see what made it worse or better. He tried different shoes, and varied his ways of standing, walking and running.

Another epiphany

Tom noticed that sitting on his hamstrings re-created the stabbing heel pain he experienced each morning on getting out of bed. Stretching his hamstrings before standing dissolved the heel pain in moments. Also, sitting on his sitz bones (*ischial tuberosities*), as opposed to his butt and thigh muscles, did not induce heel pain. This required a firm, flat chair. Rounded, heavily padded, armchairs, were the worst for this effect.

These observations are inconsistent with inflammation of the plantar fascia. Inflammation doesn't come and go like that. You can't stretch inflammation away in seconds. Tom found published research that demonstrated biomechanical (body movement) abnormalities in people with *NFP ('plantar fasciitis')*.

This led Tom to an interest in the ASTRO®, an apparatus described by the manufacturers, as:

ASTRO XO™ is a flexible exoskeleton attached to the lower leg that effectively promotes rehabilitation of ankle power and forward propulsion to treat multiple soft tissue and joint disorders that lead to gait deficiencies.

This device is designed to retrain proprioceptive behavior (more about that later). The manufacturer kindly provided Tom with an ASTRO® for him to test. He found that the device caused his foot to extend as it leaves the ground. Tom then learned to mimic this effect, while not wearing the device, with clear improvement of his *NFP ('plantar fasciitis')* symptoms. This experience provided Tom with further convincing evidence that body movement stresses were the underlying cause of *NFP ('plantar fasciitis')*, not inflammation of the plantar fascia.

This led to Tom's working hypothesis, mentioned previously, and his proposed name for the condition. Let's repeat his working hypothesis, as it's a bit of a mouthful.

Tom's Working Hypothesis

So-called plantar fasciitis, acute morning heel pain or runner's heel pain, is a progressive condition. In its early stages, it is a nociceptive (pain-causing) response to body movement stresses. This pain is a warning of worse to come, including tissue damage, if you don't change the way you move! Hence, this foot pain is nociceptive in nature. Thus, Tom recommends the name, nociceptive foot pain (NFP).

This was only a working hypothesis, requiring further research. Tom was aware that small changes in one limb can influence whole body movement. He remembered a group Feldenkrais class, in which everyone walked around, relaxed. Then the instructor asked them to grip one hand tight. The effect on movement and coordination was dramatic. The hand tension spread to the arm, then the shoulder and beyond. This self-induced tension disturbed locomotion in distinct ways.

Tom contemplated the long list of advertised treatments for *NFP ('plantar fasciitis')*. He wondered how they might each change the way one moves. He thought, *Heel injections and calf surgery would surely change my movements. Then, a roller or stretching could change the way my body works.*

How about prayer? Well, if it calmed me down, my movements would become more fluid. The same might be true of ankle magnets.

The boot in bed sure was horrible, but holding my calf tight all night made me hobble out of bed the next day. It didn't work for my heel pain, but it might for others. As would different shoes, or scraping the bottom of your feet with metal tools.

Then there's pregnancy, which sure as hell comes with modified pelvic angle, spinal stresses and body weight. Thus, pregnancy also influences body movement in a big way.

That is also true of barefoot running, which prevents heel strike and forces a low-impact style.

Is body movement the key?

Tom proceeded to apply Occam's Razor (*Among competing hypotheses, the one with the fewest assumptions should be selected*) to treatment choices for this form of heel pain.

Tom concluded that *NFP ('plantar fasciitis')* is best treated by changing the way one moves, not with expensive and dangerous heel injections. And certainly not with dangerous, expensive and irreversible surgery!

A word about proprioception

Tom continued his studies, reading what he could about body movement. He had a hunch that this was the underlying principal he was seeking. Indeed, pain can be induced by the way we move our bodies. Ever pulled your back reaching for a high shelf? Our bodies are complex machines, and they have minds of their own.

As Caroline Joy, a masseuse and expert in body physiology, says:

Proprioception refers to the body's conscious awareness of itself...

As you read this, your trunk is unconsciously adjusting as your eyes shift... your muscles perform a delicate dance of contraction and relaxation... prepared to jump into action, without conscious deliberation or direction.

The way we move is the product of a range of reflexes. These important controls adapt to our movement choices throughout our lives. When we change the way we move, we are training our proprioceptive systems.

So each muscle in our body has a mind of its own, and each of these minds thinks in a slightly different way. For instance, Tom found (with instruction from Rebecca) that you can easily relax your *psoas* muscles with your thumb. Just run your thumb down the inside of your pelvis, along the ilium (major hip bone that sticks up on either side of your hips, where you hook the belt of your pants). If this hip flexor is stressed and tense, seek the tight strand of muscle. It will respond to pressure with pain, a little more tension, and then melt away to a more relaxed state.

Tom also discovered, by accident, that you mess with your *quadratus lumborum* at your peril. Each muscle has its own character, so tread carefully.

ON BALANCE

A key aspect of the way we move is balance. Tom was now aware of the power of good balance for swimming. He wondered how balance affected walking and running, or even when getting out of bed in the morning.

He remembered watching the struggles of inexperienced swimmers. They thrash around, wasting most of their energy gasping for air. This causes them to lift their heads. This pushes their legs down, which increases the resistance (drag) of the water as they attempt to move forward. They go from kicking their legs, to lifting their heads, in an endless struggle for air.

Learn how to balance in the water and swimming becomes a delightful dance. He wondered, *does poor balance, with constant self-correction, contribute to NFP ('plantar fasciitis')? At least in some cases.*

CHAPTER EIGHT: DISEASE PROGRESSION

Where Is Your Foot Pain Going?

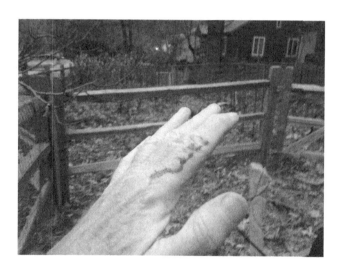

Disease

A condition of the living animal or plant body or of one of its parts that impairs normal functioning and is typically manifested by distinguishing signs and symptoms: sickness, malady. infectious diseases.

– Merriam-Webster Online Dictionary

When Tom's cat, Cat, scratched his hand, he didn't have a disease. He had a painful inconvenience.

When you have your first attack of *nociceptive foot pain* (*NFP* aka *plantar fasciitis*), you don't have a disease. You have a painful inconvenience.

In both cases, the situation can progress in a number of ways:

- Complete resolution, and no harm done.
- Partial resolution, leaving some tissue or psychological damage, of varying degrees.
- Persistence of the condition at a low level, without resolution or serious progression, with or without mild functional impairment (disease?)
- Progression with moderate to severe tissue damage and functional impairment (disease).

Tom's cat scratch

Tom's cat scratch wound may be contaminated with bacteria. This infection could progress, creating inflammation and soreness. The bacteria could proliferate and spread under Tom's skin to create more wide-spread inflammation (cellulitis). Worse they could reach lymph nodes and even enter his blood (bacteremia) to induce a wide-spread immune response due to infection of Tom's blood (septicemia). Septicemia can be fatal if it leads to septic shock.

Alternatively, how about viruses? Maybe Tom contracted *cat scratch fever*. As a veterinarian, Tom knew this, so he could watch out for the warning signs. If Tom's condition progresses to his final doom, when does he have a disease, rather and an inconvenience?

As it turned out, Tom took appropriate action. He let the wound bleed to wash out infectious organisms. He then cleaned the break in his skin with an antiseptic solution and covered it with a bandaid. Tom also kept on eye on the situation, including his lymph nodes for signs of spreading bacterial infection or viral cat scratch fever.

Don't worry, Tom's fine. The condition did not progress beyond painful inconvenience, and he still loves Cat.

PROGRESSION FROM NOCICEPTIVE FOOT PAIN

Nociceptive foot pain is unlikely to progress to a fatal disease, though it could contribute to one's demise. Chronic foot pain as a disability causes people to lose their jobs, which can lead to serious depression. Just read some plantar fasciitis stories on Facebook, if you doubt this.

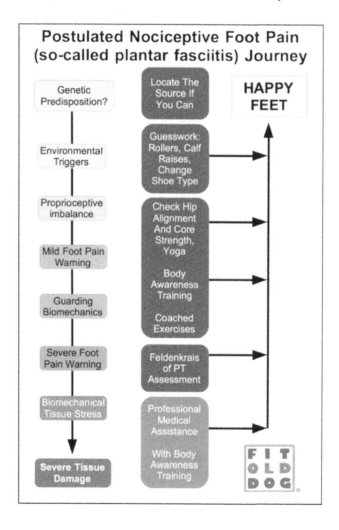

Nociceptive foot pain can progress to severe tissue damage, including:

- Degeneration, and thus weakening, of the plantar fascia and other critical support structures of the foot.
- Rupture of the plantar fascia, as occurred in Anne's case - see chapter four.
- Micro-tears in tendons and ligaments.
- Strain of the Achilles tendons.
- Even strain on the hips, leading to joint damage.
- Heel spurs.

A heel spur is a calcium deposit causing a bony protrusion on the underside of the heel bone.

– WebMD (2018)

I've made no attempt to provide a detailed review of the literature on *nociceptive foot pain* (aka *plantar fasciitis*), but here is one important report:

The authors review histologic findings from 50 cases of heel spur surgery for chronic plantar fasciitis. Findings include myxoid degeneration with fragmentation and degeneration of the plantar fascia.

(J Am Podiatr Med Assoc 93(3): 234-237, 2003).
Myxoid - resembling mucus.
The best solution is to prevent the progression. But how to do this when you don't know the cause of your *nociceptive foot pain*? Re-read chapter three, pain puzzles, for some ideas.

Tom's advice, *Look first to your hips, but keep an eye on published research. If your condition is persistent, and you suspect the risk frank tissue damage of any kind, seek professional assistance (but not a heel injection). My first choice would be a good physical therapist, but that choice is yours, as no-one can guarantee a cure. You have to be your own detective.*

It's clear that the true range of adverse consequences of chronic *nociceptive foot pain* remain to be determined.

See Chapter 10 for Tom's approach to curing *nociceptive foot pain*, before it progresses to more serious issues.

CHAPTER NINE: FOOD FOR THOUGHT

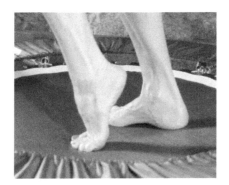

Rosemary loved her trampoline, until heel pain made it impossible.

ROSEMARY

Rosemary Glean, who lives in Washington, DC, bought Tom and Rebecca's book, and contacted them for advice. Rosemary had been diagnosed with "plantar fasciitis," but nothing was working. Tom asked Rosemary to send them a video of her standing and walking. On viewing the video, they noticed that Rosemary had collapsed arches (flat feet). This is known to be associated with *NFP ('plantar fasciitis')*.

Rebecca and Tom made a short video designed to help Rosemary correct her flat feet. This led to the following review of their work on Amazon, a few months later.

I'M ABLE TO JUMP ON MY TRAMPOLINE AGAIN.

"I ordered this book after injuring myself in April 2013. I had just finished moving all of my belongings from one apartment building to the one next door. I figured that I could handle it since it was such a short distance, but just days afterward I could barely stand without wincing. I had to stop jumping/running on my trampoline immediately, which was very difficult to adjust to the physical inactivity. I talked to my doctor and she indicated it was plantar fasciitis. I stretched and got one of those night boots, wearing it faithfully with no results. When I found this book while looking on the internet I decided to give it a try. At first I followed the basic suggestions provided and was still in pain. I decided to email him. Amazingly he emailed me back and based on my problems he and his wonderful dance teacher, Rebecca added more to the program. I have followed the protocol suggested by both as best as I can remember to on a regular basis and now I have NO PAIN when I walk. I have slowly returned to my beloved trampoline at very minimal weekly increments, starting at 30 seconds and am now up to 16 minutes, again with no pain. I appreciated that these are things that anybody, and I mean ANYBODY can do to regain the health of their feet."

– Rosemary Glean

This was a satisfying outcome. Once again, Tom thought he understood the condition. Weak calves, leading to weak arches, resulted in heel pain.
Not so fast!
Tom continued his research.

NFP ('PLANTAR FASCIITIS') OCCURS IN MULTIPLE LOCATIONS ON THE SOLE OF THE FOOT

Based on his own experience, data from fellow athletes and reports on Facebook, Tom made a map of foot pains he considered similar in nature to *NFP ('plantar fasciitis')*.

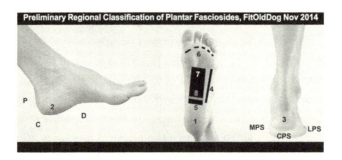

Key:

1 = sole of heel
2 = medial heel
3 = posterior heel (proximal insertion)
4 = lateral margin of sole
5 = posterior margin of sole of heel ('central' or posterior distal insertion point)
6 = anterior extremity of plantar region (distal distal insertion points)
7 = diffuse plantar region of sole
8 = zone of tearing (Tom felt this once and thought, "never again, please!")
P = proximal with respect to long axis of the body from the head
C = central region of the heel
D = distal with respect to the long axis of the body from the head
MPS = medial parasagittal
CPS = central parasagittal
LPS = lateral parasagittal.

Tom is still of the opinion that hip strength, alignment, and movements play major roles in most cases of the condition. It's clear that single-leg calf raises provide significant strength training, especially to core muscles in and around the pelvis.

There is some published research on the relationship between *NFP ('plantar fasciitis')* and nociceptive pain. Tom thinks this would be a fruitful area to investigate. One clinical study (McMillan, 2012) demonstrated that any improvement from corticosteroid injections into the plantar fascia only lasted about four weeks. Not worth the risk, in Tom's opinion.

The single-leg calf raises, mentioned in Tom's first blog post, was the subject of a small study in Sweden (Rathleff et al., 2014). These researchers reported that, this "High-load strength training may aid in a quicker reduction in pain and improvements in function."

Tom's Research Stumbles along

Tom continued to scratch his head about the mechanisms of *NFP ('plantar fasciitis')*. Everyday, he read of new cases. With all those survey data in his files, Tom wondered whether useful patterns were hidden there. This is where his previous life as a scientist came in handy.

Many years ago, Tom ran a large molecular biology lab, equipped with lots of wonderful, expensive tools. One of these tools, clustering software, was used to look for patterns in massive data sets, which contained millions of numbers. In minutes, patterns would emerge, revealing what was going on in diseased tissues.

Tom applied this approach to some of his *NFP ('plantar fasciitis')* survey data, derived from 237 individual survey responses from *NFP ('plantar fasciitis')* sufferers. This survey used twenty selected *NFP ('plantar fasciitis')* treatments. First, he converted these data to binary format (1, 0, -1, blank). He then used clustering freeware, *Cluster* and *Java Treeview*, to analyze these data. Clustering statistics revealed two groups or subsets of people diagnosed with *NFP ('plantar fasciitis')*. Cases that tend to respond to one or more of the treatments, and those people that tend not to respond.

This work demonstrated clear heterogeneity between *NFP ('plantar fasciitis')* sufferers. Further clustering failed to reveal information that Tom was able to interpret with his statistical skills. Such studies need to be extended in order to guide subgroups of people with *NFP ('plantar fasciitis')* towards an optimal treatment strategy.

Remote Sensation Mapping

Tom doesn't have a lab, or staff, or millions of dollars worth of equipment, anymore. He has his dwindling retirement funds, and whatever stuff he can find around the house or in his mind.

Tom thought, *Nociceptive foot pain almost certainly comes from upstream. It's a warning of a movement problem somewhere. Are there sensory links between different regions of my feet and these regions of my body? If these links exist, they could provide clues about where the mechanical problems lie, with respect to the source of the nociception.*

Tom reached for a coat hanger.

The information in the following image was created using a carefully crafted tool, with which Tom gently stroked the bottom of his feet and listened for sensations in his body.

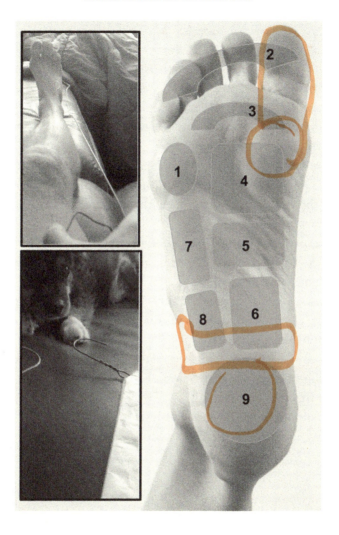

Mapping was thus carried out using this highly sophisticated neurostimulator (lower left: construction materials, guarded by Scooter, Tom's lovely little, old, deaf and blind, but happy dog; upper left: completed neurostimulator tool). The signal was Tom's perception of a sensory link between the stimulated part of his foot and other regions of his body.

IMPORTANT NOTE: *All linked sensations, except for those from foot area 1, were ipsilateral (same side).*

When an area of Tom's right foot was gently stroked with the probe tip, a non-painful link sensation was observed to project from the foot area *numbered, to: (1) Tom's left, damaged shoulder, (2) right upper back, (3) right middle back, (4) right lower back, where you get hip flexor (psoas) pain, (5) right lower back, near tail bone, (6) over right side of tail bone, (7) right hips, region of pyriformis and lateral gluts, (8) same as 7 but deeper, (9) really complicated, on right pelvic floor, needing more detailed mapping.* It will take time and more sophisticated neurophysiological equipment than a coat hanger to work that one out.

Tom was fascinated by the complexity of sensations from the heel, thinking, "Maybe the sensory receptors in the heel project to many areas of the body, causing it to be the most common site of *NFP* ('*plantar fasciitis*') pain."

This experiment turned out to be pretty interesting, to Tom. It's how one does research: You go down one blind alley after another until you find a meaningful answer.

For instance, look at areas 7 and 8 in the figure. Tom noticed that in the past, tightness in his hips was often associated with pain in these regions of his feet. This was especially true for tightness involving the *glut minimus* and *pyriformis* muscles. The neurostimulator sensory link observation fits this pain experience.

But is this real science, junk science or BS?

Who knows? Tom isn't sure, but it does provide food for thought.

CHAPTER 10: TOM'S NFP TREATMENT STRATEGY

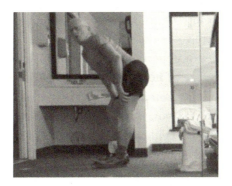

Tom learns how to stretch his hips to reduce the risk of NFP ('plantar fasciitis') and other problems. You can access the video on the FitOldDog YouTube channel.

Body movement modification or dangerous heel injections? Research will tell us who's right in the end. Here's Tom's recommended *NFP ('plantar fasciitis')* treatment approach, in a nutshell:

1. **Be sure of your diagnosis**. If necessary, consult a medical professional, as there are many causes of heel pain. If it's most severe on getting out of bed in the morning, and fades

during the day, only to return the next morning, it's probably *NFP (plantar fasciitis)*. Remember, *NFP (plantar fasciitis)* can occur in other regions of the foot, and this strategy is still appropriate. Consult a physician if you're in doubt, but this can be costly, and potentially misleading. Alternatively, you could consult a body movement expert or sports massage therapist. This is truly detective work, and you are the detective.

2. **Let go of the assumption** that the problem is where the pain is.
3. **Keep a diary**. This will become your baseline or foundation. Even if you fix your pain, it can come back for the same or a different reason. We forget critical details, so write it all down.
4. **Use a coat hanger** or ask a friend to gently touch the sole of your foot in an attempt to track the source of your pain back to your hips or elsewhere, as described in chapter nine. Once you determine the source, it's a matter of relaxing tense muscles or undertaking realignment work.
5. **Become aware of how you move.** This includes sitting, standing, walking, running or other activities you enjoy.
6. **Change the way you move.** You could use a different shoe type. Take a Feldenkrais lesson. Look at your stance in the mirror and change it. You could even try smiling as you walk around. Skipping, from time to time, might do the trick. It's hard to be unhappy when you skip. Just being aware of how you move will change it to some extent. Then combine your choice with the following:
7. **Stretch** (lengthen) selected muscle groups, especially hamstrings and hips. Use active-isolated stretching, rollers or a tennis ball to release tight muscles. Remember, it's a conversation with your body, not something you do to your body, as explained in one of the FitOldDog YouTube videos.
8. **Strengthen** selected muscle groups, especially arch machinery, which includes feet, calves, thighs and hips. This is also addressed in a FitOldDog YouTube Video. Single-leg

calf raises are highly recommended, as they strengthen pelvic muscles, a common source of *NFP ('plantar fasciitis')*. Yoga, Gyrokinesis® and Continuum, are also a valuable techniques for both strengthening and realigning your body, especially your hips. Take care not to overtrain, making all changes gradually.

9. **Realign** misaligned tissues, with especial attention to hips. It took an osteopathic doctor to realign Tom's pelvis. This was one of the underlying causes of his second case of *NFP ('plantar fasciitis')*. You can seek the help of a physical therapist, massage therapist or other health professional, to help you with soft tissue issues. Again, Yoga can be an effective approach.
10. **Learn how to listen to your body.** Turn off music and other distractions and look inward.
11. **Don't assume that your doctor knows best** when it comes to *NFP ('plantar fasciitis')*. No one knows your body better than you.
12. **It's detective work** so hang in there. If you're stuck, write to the author and ask for ideas (olddogintraining@gmail.com).

EPILOGUE

Tom's Onto Something!

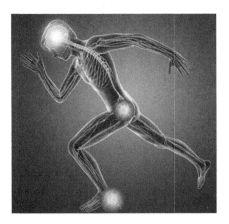

The experience with the neurostimulator allowed Tom to track down the source of another, more recent, dose of *NFP (plantar fasciitis)* heel pain. This permitted him to fix the problem in minutes, by revealing the source of the pain. It went like this:

Tom ran 10 miles. It was his first fairly long run of his current marathon training plan, on a pretty tough trail. Then he did only minimal post-run stretching and proceeded to sit on his hamstrings (bad idea!) for a couple of hours. He was busy writing on his computer.

When Tom got up and put weight on his feet, there it was. Stabbing pain in the center of his right heel.

Tom thought, *Um! Another opportunity to do some NFP ('plantar fasciitis') research. I'll get out the old neurostimulator. No, I'll make a new one, with an improved design."* It was still made from a wire coat hanger, but this prototype's end was rounded instead of sharp. It worked nicely.

First Tom checked area 1 (see diagram in chapter 9). He sees this as a critical test of the method. Yep, still reached his opposite hip. Then he tested the other regions of the sole of his affect right foot, to be sure all was on track. Finally, Tom came to his real interpretational challenge, the right heel (area 9).

Tom already knew that his heel is the most challenging region of all, in terms of sensing the location of feelings in his body that are linked to the sole his foot.

Brushing his heel immediately revealed areas of tension or discomfort in the same leg, in his medial hamstrings, hip flexors (*psoas* and *iliacus*), and other hip muscles (*gluteus lateralis* and *minimus*, and hip rotators, especially the *pyriformis,* an old injury friend). It turns out that his right hip was extremely tight.

So Tom carried out one of his standard stretching routines for these muscles. The heel discomfort faded in minutes.

Looks as though Tom is onto something.

RESULT:

A coat hanger may be a better therapeutic tool than heel injections or Strayer calf surgery craziness.

POST-SCRIPT

A metaphor for NFP ('plantar fasciitis')

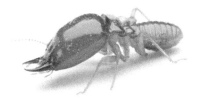

TERMITES?

Tom's sitting with a flashlight, in muddy water up to his waist, and he's wondering!

Here I am, in the cobwebby crawl space of our house, it's due to go on the market. An inspector found termite damage. Half the staircase is being replaced. Good thing we have a termite contract.

But why termites?

It's a pretty new, cooky cutter house. Affordable because of its remoteness. Furthermore, Tom's not a guy who likes to work on houses, or cars for that matter. He can, but he prefers to do other things.

Well, termites like dark and damp. Into the crawl space he went.

Cobwebs, dirt, a muddy floor. No sign of standing water, but plenty of damp. This house faced the road. In front was a long lawn that sloped up, away from the house. Tom thought water from the lawn must be draining into the crawl space when it rains.

Tom decided to go under there during a rain storm. Within minutes, the next storm arrived, dumping enough water into that crawl space to play *Pooh Sticks*. A large pool (*heel pain*) was forming against the cinder-block wall at the back of the house. Tom thought the problem came from the house being on a piece of sloping land. Water flow was worse on the right than the left, but the biggest pool accumulated in the center.

Being human, Tom rushed for a solution. It's how humans evolved. Rustling grass? A tiger or the wind. Those who waited to find out were deleted from the gene pool.

Go figure!

If water is getting into the crawl space, causing termites, I need to remove the water. **It's obvious.** Off Tom goes to the hardware store, to buy a sump pump (*have a heel injection!*). This is a standard approach to water in a cellar (*pain in your heel!*).

He reads the instructions, and hunts for a place to hook up the power, following code. That done, he starts to dig. This creates a sizable pit, where water has been pooling during rain storms. It's a muddy job. He sits with the pump, placed it in a bucket at the center of the muddy hole.

Then it starts to rain again. A heavy storm. Before he knows it, Tom's in water up to his waist.

The light finally came on.

Wait a minute! Where is this water coming from? It arrives too fast to be the lawn. Hell, I know enough about grass and fluid mechanics to figure that one out. Damn, it must be coming from the roof. But how? Gutters, downspouts, and drains carry roof water away from the house.

Curiouser and curiouser!

Tom decides it's time to get some advice. He calls his handyman, Karl, who tells him to check the downspouts.

Tom starts to dig around the base of the right hand downspout, where it enters the ground. He removes the mulch, to find that the downspout isn't connected to the drain pipe. Storm water is flooding the ground around the drainage pipe.

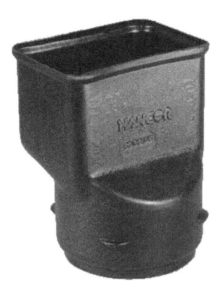

Wait a minute. The builder "forgot" to install a downspout adapter! A simple connector, costing about $1.

> *For want of a nail a shoe was lost.*
> *For want of a shoe a horse was lost.*
> *For want of a horse a king was lost.*
> *For want of a king a kingdom was lost.*

Thousands of dollars of repair for the Termite Company. A delayed house sale, a wasted sump pump purchase. All for a piece of plastic costing $1.

Tom realized that this was the perfect metaphor for *NFP (plantar fasciitis)*. Like a missing downspout adapter, one tight muscle in your pelvis can lead to years of misery and expense.

Observe the problem closely, then question the obvious, and find a way to fix it!

A PLEA

The author's plea to the medical community is that they put down their cortisone-charged syringes. That they stop cutting up people's calves to cure persistent so-called plantar fasciitis. That they invest significant time and research dollars in the understanding of *NFP ('plantar fasciitis')*, as a road to reliable and safe treatment protocols.

ACKNOWLEDGMENTS

Thanks are due to hundreds of people who helped Tom on his journey of discovery, from the author's mom to Moshe Feldenkrais. They can't all be listed, but they know who they are. Thanks are due Debbie Young, of the ALLi Member forum. Debbie led the author to Joanna Penn, of the Creative Penn, who told him about Vellum book publishing software. This made designing the book so much easier. The encouraging comments on Tom's front cover design, by Andy Fleishman, an artist and friend, is also much appreciated. This cover was created using an image and copyright purchased from Shutter-Stock, combined with Apple's Pages and Adobe Photoshop software. Finally, thanks so much to Lisa Carl for her excellent and constructive editing.

ABOUT THE AUTHOR

Dr. Kevin Thomas Morgan is a retired veterinary pathologist and research scientist. He now works on ways to help older people keep going, to enjoy every day they are lucky enough to have. He does this by writing books, creating instructional videos, and giving entertaining talks. His current interests include reading and learning to write. He enjoys solving problems to help people in pain. Kevin is an avid vegetable gardener and vegan. Some of his work is designed to help people who, like himself, have aortic disease. He enjoys friends and family, and not being dead for as long as possible.

OTHER BOOKS BY THE AUTHOR

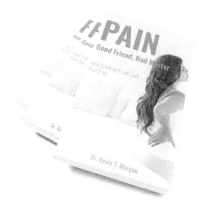

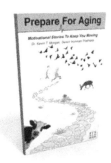

OTHER BOOKS BY THE AUTHOR

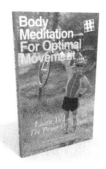

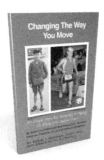

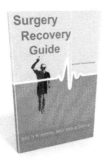

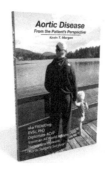

NEWSLETTER SIGNUP LINK

Old Dogs in Training LLC newsletters are published once or twice per month. They relate to preparing for aging, living with vascular disease, including aortic aneurysm, safe exercise for older people, nociceptive foot pain aka plantar fasciitis, and other subjects that interest the author, with respect to enjoying our later years, actively.

Oh! From time to time recommended books are also highlighted, as the author loves to read.

You can sign up for the newsletter on the authors blog, AthleteWithStent.Com.

COPYRIGHT AND DISCLAIMER

Copyright and Medical Disclaimer © 2018

Kevin T. Morgan, Old Dogs in Training, LLC.

All rights reserved. This book may not be reproduced, in whole or in part, in any form or by any means electronic or mechanical, including photocopying, recording or by any information storage and retrieval system now known or hereafter invented, without written permission from the author, Kevin Thomas Morgan, aka FitOldDog.

Copyrights for images, not the original property of the author, were purchased from, and copyrights are filed with, ShutterStock, Inc.

LIMIT OF LIABILITY AND DISCLAIMER

This document is based on the author's experience and has been created to provide information and guidance about the subject matter covered. Every effort has been made to make it as accurate as possible. Website links and content can change at any time. If a link is nonfunctional, please contact the author. The author shall have neither liability nor responsibility to any person or entity with respect to any loss, damage or injury caused or alleged to be caused directly or indirectly by the information covered in this book, or by decisions made based upon this book.

TRADEMARKS

Any trademarks, service marks, product names or named features are assumed to be the property of their respective owners, and are used for reference only.

SHARING THIS DOCUMENT

I politely ask that you please respect my work by not donating or reselling this book. I appreciate your respect of this creative process.

MEDICAL DISCLAIMER

As a veterinarian, the author does not provide medical advice to human animals. Before you undertake any exercise program, consult your medical advisers. Undertaking activities discussed by the author does not mean that he endorses your activity, which is clearly your decision and responsibility. Be careful and sensible, please.

FitOldDog, Old Dogs in Training, LLC.